Table of Contents

Introduction

Herpes Simplex Virus is a skin infection. It is of two types- Herpes type 1 and Herpes Type 2. Herpes type 1 is also called oral herpes and herpes type 2 is also known as genital herpes. You can fight with herpes with strong immune system. Generally, doctors recommend anti-viral such as acyclovir, famcyclovir and Valacyclovir but they don't know about any alternative of these supplements. These medicines can only help you for a short period of time as they have so many side-effects like headache, nausea and anxiety. Anti-viral can also damage your immune system. These medicines cannot cure your herpes. There are many options to cure herpes naturally. You can get rid of herpes with natural cure. Most of the people say that there is no cure for herpes. But Dr. Sebi has found the cure for herpes. He is not a doctorate doctor or a degree holder. But he claims that he has been found the cure for a non-curable skin infection, herpes. Not only herpes, he has cured many other non-curable diseases such as HIV-aids, cancer and many more. Many people claim that he has cured their incurable illness. A person claims that Dr. Sebi cured his HIV in just 2months. He cured diseases like HIV and herpes with natural and organic remedies. He believed that nature can cure any disease. Nature is your true friend in the battle of herpes. It can help you to get rid of herpes. Natural resources such as Aloe Vera, Olive Oil, lemon balm and lysine are proved resources to help in the treatment of herpes. So, instead of going for medicines prescribed by your doctor, go for natural ways to get rid of your herpes infection. There are no side-effects of using natural home remedies and it will also help you to cure herpes permanently. According to Western medicine, there is no cure for herpes. However, Dr Sebi claims to have cured herpes in addition to other incurable diseases such as HIV, Lupus, Cancer, etc. This book contains information on Dr. Sebi diet and it cure for HIV and herpes.

Who Is Dr. Sebi

Dr. Sebi born Alfredo Bowman came to the United States as a self-educated man who was diagnosed with asthma, diabetes, impotency, and obesity. After unsuccessful treatments with conventional doctors and chemical-based medications, Sebi soon found himself the lead to an herbalist in Mexico. Finding great healing success from all his ailments, he began creating capsules, powders, tonics, teas, and salves that the supreme court classified as "natural vegetation cell food". These compounds are geared for inter-cellular cleansing and food for the cells that make up the human body. Dr. Sebi has dedicated over 30 years of his life to developing a unique methodology that he obtained through years of observational and first-hand knowledge.

Dr. Sebi Diet

Dr. Sebi believed the Western approach to disease to be ineffective. He held that mucus and acidity — rather bacteria and viruses, for example — caused disease. A main theory behind the diet is that disease can only survive in acidic environments. The aim of the diet is to achieve an alkaline state in the body in order to prevent or eradicate disease. The diet's official website sells botanical remedies that it claims will detoxify the body. The site links to no research that would support its claims about health benefits. It does note that the Food and Drug Administration (FDA) have not evaluated the statements. Those behind the site acknowledge that they are not medical doctors and do not intend the site's content to replace medical advice.

Dr. Sebi: Food Therapy

Dr. Sebi connects the dots between physical/mental disease and diet. A malnourished person, someone deficient in vitamins and minerals, has a brain that is breaking down resulting in erratic thinking and ultimately harmful actions. When the body has what it needs, it is tranquil. Healing the gut by removing toxins is linked to healing the brain. Toxins are removed from an alkaline diet that are free from acid-based foods. Happiness is compromised when the body is acidic. When the body is highly acidic, instability, insanity, discontent, and violence occur.

Follow the model of life: nature. From nature, we get phosphates, carbonates, iodides, and bromides. These are considered by biochemistry as food. If we eat proper foods, we don't need nutritionists. Elephants, bears and all animals don't have nutritionists. Foods based on starch are scientifically known as carbonic acid. It creates a reaction that produces sulfides which rob the body of oxygen. To obtain an electric body, we must eat electric foods. Electric foods assist digestion and assimilation. Healing covers every aspect of man. Healing brings peace and there can be no peace unless there is wellness in the body.

How To Follow The Diet

Dr. Sebi's nutritional guide includes a number of rules, such as:

• Only eat foods listed in the guide.

• Drink 1 gallon of natural spring water daily.

• Avoid animal products, hybrid foods, and alcohol.

• Avoid using a microwave, which will "kill your food."

• Avoid canned and seedless fruits.

Foods To Eat

Dr. Sebi's nutrition guide details specific foods allowed on the diet, including:

• Fruits: apples, cantaloupe, currants, dates, figs, elderberries, papayas, berries, peaches, soft jelly coconuts, pears, plums, seeded key limes, mangoes, prickly pears, seeded melons, Latin or West Indies soursop, tamarind

• Vegetables: avocado, bell peppers, cactus flower, chickpeas, cucumber, dandelion greens, kale, lettuce (except iceberg), mushrooms (except shiitake), okra, olives, sea vegetables, squash, tomatoes (only cherry and plum), zucchini

• Grains: fonio, amaranth, Khorasan wheat (kamut), rye, wild rice, spelt, teff, quinoa

• Nuts and Seeds: Brazil nuts, hemp seeds, raw sesame seeds, raw tahini butter, walnuts

• Oils: avocado oil, coconut oil (uncooked), grapeseed oil, hempseed oil, olive oil (uncooked), sesame oil

• Herbal teas: elderberry, chamomile, fennel, tila, burdock, ginger, raspberry

• Spices: oregano, basil, cloves, bay leaf, dill, sweet basil, achiote, cayenne, habanero, tarragon, onion powder, sage, pure sea salt, thyme, powdered granulated seaweed, pure agave syrup, date sugar

In addition to tea, you are allowed to drink water. Plus, you may eat permitted grains in the form of pasta, cereal, bread, or flour. However, any food leavened with yeast or baking powder is banned.

Foods To Avoid

Any foods that are not included in the Dr. Sebi nutrition guide are not permitted, such as:

• canned fruit or vegetables

- seedless fruit

- eggs

- dairy

- fish

- red meat

- poultry

- soy products

- processed food, including take-out or restaurant food

- fortified foods

- wheat

- sugar (besides date sugar and agave syrup)

- alcohol

- yeast or foods risen with yeast

- foods made with baking powder

Furthermore, many vegetables, fruits, grains, nuts, and seeds are banned on the diet. Only foods listed in the guide may be eaten.

What Dr. Sebi Says About Brain Health

The brain needs oxygen and mucus blocks oxygen to the brain by causing inflammation. Mucus must be removed from the brain so that it can heal and oxygen can flow through. The brain is an electrical organ and the only organ in the body that produces electricity. Electricity is produced through the friction of copper and carbon. The brain is made up of these two minerals and it is the center of producing motion in the body. The nervous system carries electrical currents formed in the brain throughout the body to cause movement. When consuming acidic foods like dairy and starch, the brain suffers first-thought patterns change and the body stresses. Iron is the mineral that carries oxygen to the brain. When the body is low in iron, the brain cannot receive oxygen. Dr. Sebi recommends "electric food"- foods that have iron as a dominant mineral and are alkaline.

Oxygen

The benefit: Oxygen sustains life. It is the unlimited essential supply of the air we breathe. It is necessary because it removes toxins from the blood and cells while also repairing damaged tissue caused by inflammation. This element is also responsible for healthy sleep cycles resulting in clearer thinking and alertness.

What to eat: Alkaline water with a pH of 7 and above. Foods that increase oxygen to the brain are avocados, watercress, organic apples, berries, dates, mango, and papaya.

Meal tip: A smoothie would be the easiest way to combine a large combination of these ingredients such as a blend of apples, berries, dates, and mango with hemp milk.

Phenolic Compounds

The benefits: Fruits and vegetables contain phenolic compounds that are plant metabolites whose function is to produce energy. These metabolites have been linked to protecting against oxidative damaging diseases (heart disease, stroke, and cancers). It's suggested that diets rich in phenolic compounds may have preventative effects on the development of brain diseases like alzheimer's and dementia. Phenolic compounds have also been found to have potent antioxidative properties for regulating inflammatory responses that support brain function.

What to eat: Foods rich in phenolic compounds include: Olive oil, blackberries, blueberries, burdock root(tea), cherries, kiwis, seeded grapes, apples, onions, turmeric and kale.

Meal tip: A good way to incorporate these ingredients is a kale salad rubbed with olive oil, turmeric, and sea salt with added avocado, garbanzo beans, onions and a cup of burdock root tea.

Vitamins A, C, B6 & Iron

The benefits: Vitamins A, C, B6 and iron are all antioxidant vitamins and minerals that have big impacts, which protect our health by fighting infections and free radicals in the environment. This is critical for our overall health, particularly mood and mental health. Additionally, there is evidence that shows that the lack of these antioxidants and minerals may lead to anemia which occurs when there are not enough healthy red blood cells in the body. Iron is a magnetic mineral that pulls other minerals to it. A body with a healthy amount of iron attracts other minerals.

What to eat: Foods rich in vitamin A: Winter squash, turnip greens, sweet red pepper, mango, cantaloupe, seeded watermelon, papaya, wild rice, quinoa, spelt

• Foods rich in vitamin C: Guava, parsley, key limes, cherry tomatoes, lettuce

• Foods rich in vitamin B6: Chickpeas, burro bananas, walnuts, brazil nuts, raisins,

• Dried peaches, tahini butter, hemp seeds, and dandelion greens are large sources of iron.

Meal tip: An excellent meal full of these vitamins and minerals might include baked falafel topped with tahini butter, a green salad with romaine lettuce, cherry tomatoes, and red bell pepper, and a side of roasted squash.

Tips For Sticking To The Diet

Like any other diet you try, this one will take time and effort! While it may be difficult at first, your body will slowly get used to this new way of eating. You will begin to feel more energized as you eliminate all the bad foods you may have consumed in the past. Down below are a few suggestions and guidelines to follow to make this the most enjoyable experience possible.

• Drink Plenty of Water: According to Bowman, people should be drinking at least a gallon of water per day. This is essential to making this alkaline diet work to the best of its ability. Alfredo recommends natural spring water as opposed to water softeners or water from a reverse osmosis system. Other health organizations and nutritional experts suggest a gallon of water per day too. Keep in mind that water removes waste from the body while assisting in the absorption of nutrients and cushioning joints and organs.

• Be Emotionally and Mentally Prepared: It is extremely likely that you have formed some strong habits eating certain types of foods daily that may make it very hard to break or change your diet. Your family and friends may also become a hindrance when trying to carry out this diet. Before beginning this plan, spend some time thinking about why you want to change your eating and the obstacles, both mental and emotional, that you will face.

• Don't Give up Snacks: Yes, you heard right. While you do not have to give up snacks, you do have to snack the right way. This means instead of reaching for a bag of potato chips, eat a piece of fruit or create snacks based on the recommended nutritional guide.

• Review the Approved Foods: Do your best not to stray from the list of approved foods as it can hinder your results. While it may seem too difficult at first to eat from the selected list, you'll soon find it's easier than thought especially if you are prepared mentally.

• Add Whole Foods to Your Diet: Do your best to substitute packaged foods with whole foods in your diet on a regular basis. You want to avoid packaged foods because they are full of additives, which can be very addictive especially since many have refined sugar that causes food cravings.

• Cooking is Essential: You will quickly find that it's necessary to cook when trying this diet. The guides offer alkaline food recipes to make this process easier. His guides walk you step by step through each alkaline meal. After you begin preparing your own meals, you'll see how you can take your favorite dishes and prepare them using approved ingredients.

Sample Menu
Here is a three-day sample menu on the Dr. Sebi diet.

Day 1

- Breakfast: 2 banana-spelt pancakes with agave syrup

- Snack: 1 cup (240 ml) of green juice smoothie made with cucumbers, kale, apples, and ginger

- Lunch: kale salad with tomatoes, onions, avocado, dandelion greens, and chickpeas with olive oil and basil dressing

- Snack: herbal tea with fruit

- Dinner: vegetable and wild-rice stir-fry

Day 2

- Breakfast: shake made with water, hemp seeds, bananas, and strawberries

- Snack: blueberry muffins made with blueberries, pure coconut milk, agave syrup, sea salt, oil, and teff and spelt flour

- Lunch: homemade pizza using a spelt-flour crust, Brazil-nut cheese, and your choice of vegetables

- Snack: tahini butter on rye bread with sliced red peppers on the side

• Dinner: chickpea burger with tomato, onion, and kale on spelt-flour flatbread

Day 3

• Breakfast: cooked quinoa with agave syrup, peaches, and pure coconut milk

• Snack: chamomile tea, seeded grapes, and sesame seeds

• Lunch: spelt-pasta salad with chopped vegetables and an olive oil and key lime dressing

• Snack: a smoothie made with mango, banana, and pure coconut milk

• Dinner: hearty vegetable soup using mushrooms, red peppers, zucchini, onions, kale, spices, water, and powdered seaweed

Benefits Of Dr Sebi Diet

There is a lack of any scientific evidence to support the Dr. Sebi diet. However, research indicates that a plant-based diet can benefit health. There are also risks to consider, which we discuss in the next section. Some health benefits of plant-based diets may include:

• Weight loss — a 2015 study concluded that a vegan diet resulted in more weight loss than other, less restrictive diets. Participants lost up to 7.5% of body weight after 6 months on a vegan diet.

• Appetite control — a 2016 study in young male participants found that they felt fuller and more satisfied after eating a plant-based meal containing peas and beans than a meal containing meat.

• Altering the microbiome -— the term "microbiome" collectively refers to the microorganisms in the gut. A 2019 study found that a plant-based diet could alter the microbiome favorably, leading to less risk of disease. However, confirming this will require more research.

• Reduced risk of disease — a 2017 review concluded that a plant-based diet may reduce the risk of coronary heart disease by 40% and the risk of developing metabolic syndrome and type 2 diabetes by half.

The Dr. Sebi diet encourages people to eat whole foods and avoids processed foods. A study from 2017 found that reducing the intake of processed food would improve the nutritional quality of the general diet in the United States.

Downsides Of The Dr. Sebi Diet

Keep in mind that there are several drawbacks to this diet.

Highly restrictive

A major downside of Dr. Sebi's diet is that it restricts large groups of food, such as all animal products, wheat, beans, lentils, and many types of vegetables and fruit. In fact, it's so strict that it only allows specific types of fruit. For example, you're allowed to eat cherry or plum tomatoes but not other varieties like beefsteak or roma tomatoes. Moreover, following such a restrictive diet is not enjoyable and may lead to a negative relationship with food, especially since this diet vilifies foods that are not listed in the nutrition guide. Finally, this diet encourages other negative behaviors, such as using supplements to achieve fullness. Given that supplements are not a major source of calories, this claim further drives unhealthy eating patterns.

Lacks protein and other essential nutrients

The foods listed in Dr. Sebi's nutrition guide can be an excellent source of nutrition. However, none of the permitted foods are good sources of protein, an essential nutrient for skin structure, muscle growth, and the production of enzymes and hormones. Only walnuts, Brazil nuts, sesame seeds, and hemp seeds are permitted, which aren't great sources of protein. For example, 1/4 cup (25 grams) of walnuts and 3 tbsp (30 grams) of hemp seeds provide 4 grams and 9 grams of protein, respectively. To meet your daily protein needs, you would need to eat extremely large portions of these foods. Though foods in this diet are high in certain nutrients, such as beta carotene, potassium, and vitamins C and E, they're low in omega-3, iron, calcium, and vitamins D and B12, which are common nutrients of concern for those following a strictly plant-based diet. Dr. Sebi's website states that certain ingredients in his supplements are proprietary and not listed. This is concerning, as it's unclear which nutrients you're getting and how much, making it difficult to know whether you'll meet your daily nutrient needs.

Not based on real science

One of the biggest concerns with Dr. Sebi's diet approach is the lack of scientific evidence to support it. He states that the foods and supplements in his diet control acid production in your body. However, the human body strictly regulates acid-base balance to keep blood pH levels between 7.36 and 7.44, naturally making your body slightly alkaline. In rare cases, such as ketoacidosis from diabetes, blood pH can go out of this range. This can be fatal without immediate medical attention. Finally, research has shown that your diet may slightly and temporarily change your urine pH but not blood pH. Therefore, following Dr. Sebi's diet will not make your body more alkaline.

Adopting An Alkaline Diet Via Dr. Sebi

Dr Sebi's methodology involved using a natural alkaline plant food diet and herbs to alkalize the body to return the alkaline body back to a state of homeostasis. The diet consisted of only natural alkaline vegetables, fruits, nuts, alkaline grains, and legumes, which would alkalize and remove mucus from the body. Along with the diet he also used natural alkaline herbs to clean the body's cells on the cellular, and intra-cellular level. The alkaline diet is based on the premise that disease can only exist in an acidic environment. The body works to maintain a slightly alkaline 7.4 pH environment in the blood. View what happens when the blood becomes acidic. The blood is the point of equilibrium for homeostasis and when the body becomes too acidic the body will borrow alkaline minerals and compounds from bones and fluids through the body to put into the blood to keep its pH stable. This jeopardize the health of different areas of the body and lead to the development of disease.

HIV

HIV is a virus that damages the immune system. The immune system helps the body fight off infections. Untreated HIV infects and kills CD4 cells, which are a type of immune cell called T cells. Over time, as HIV kills more CD4 cells, the body is more likely to get various types of infections and cancers. HIV is transmitted through bodily fluids that include:

• blood

• semen

• vaginal and rectal fluids

• breast milk

The virus doesn't spread in air or water, or through casual contact. HIV is a lifelong condition and currently there is no cure, although many scientists are working to find one. However, with medical care, including treatment called antiretroviral therapy, it's possible to manage HIV and live with the virus for many years. Without treatment, a person with HIV is likely to develop a serious condition called AIDS. At that point, the immune system is too weak to fight off other diseases and infections. Untreated, life expectancy with AIDS is about three years. With antiretroviral therapy, HIV can be well-controlled and life expectancy can be nearly the same as someone who has not contracted HIV. It's estimated that 1.1 million Americans are currently living with HIV. Of those people, 1 in 5 don't know they have the virus. HIV can cause changes throughout the body.

AIDS

AIDS is a disease that can develop in people with HIV. It's the most advanced stage of HIV. But just because a person has HIV doesn't mean they'll develop AIDS. HIV kills CD4 cells. Healthy adults generally have a CD4 count of 500 to 1,500 per cubic millimeter. A person with HIV whose CD4 count falls below 200 per cubic millimeter will be diagnosed with AIDS. A person can also be diagnosed with AIDS if they have HIV and develop an opportunistic infection or cancer that's rare in people who don't have

HIV. An opportunistic infection, such as pneumonia, is one that takes advantage of a unique situation, such as HIV. Untreated, HIV can progress to AIDS within a decade. There's no cure for AIDS, and without treatment, life expectancy after diagnosis is about three years. This may be shorter if the person develops a severe opportunistic illness. However, treatment with antiretroviral drugs can prevent AIDS from developing. If AIDS does develop, it means that the immune system is severely compromised. It's weakened to the point where it can no longer fight off most diseases and infections. That makes the person vulnerable to a wide range of illnesses, including:

• pneumonia

• tuberculosis

• oral thrush, a fungal infection in the mouth or throat

• cytomegalovirus (CMV), a type of herpes virus

• cryptococcal meningitis, a fungal infection in the brain

• toxoplasmosis, a brain infection caused by a parasite

• cryptosporidiosis, an infection caused by an intestinal parasite

• cancer, including Kaposi's sarcoma (KS) and lymphoma

The shortened life expectancy linked with untreated AIDS isn't a direct result of the syndrome itself. Rather, it's a result of the diseases and complications that arise from having an immune system weakened by AIDS.

HIV And AIDS: The Connection

To develop AIDS, a person has to have contracted HIV. But having HIV doesn't necessarily mean that someone will develop AIDS. Cases of HIV progress through three stages:

• stage 1: acute stage, the first few weeks after transmission

• stage 2: clinical latency, or chronic stage

• stage 3: AIDS

As HIV lowers the CD4 cell count, the immune system weakens. A typical adult's CD4 count is 500 to 1,500 per cubic millimeter. A person with a count below 200 is considered to have AIDS. How quickly a case of HIV progresses through the chronic stage varies significantly from person to person. Without treatment, it can last up to a decade before advancing to AIDS. With treatment, it can last indefinitely. There is no cure for HIV, but it can be controlled. People with HIV often have a near-normal lifespan with early treatment with antiretroviral therapy. Along those same lines, there's technically no cure for AIDS. However, treatment can increase a person's CD4 count to the point where they're considered to no longer have AIDS. (This point is a count of 200 or higher.) Also, treatment can typically help manage opportunistic infections. HIV and AIDS are related, but they're not the same thing.

HIV Transmission

Anyone can contract HIV. The virus is transmitted in bodily fluids that include:

• blood

• semen

• vaginal and rectal fluids

• breast milk

Some of the way HIV is spread from person to person include:

• through vaginal or anal sex — the most common route of transmission, especially among men who have sex with men

• by sharing needles, syringes, and other items for injection drug use

• by sharing tattoo equipment without sterilizing it between uses

• during pregnancy, labor, or delivery from a woman to her baby

• during breastfeeding

• through "pre-mastication," or chewing a baby's food before feeding it to them

• through exposure to the blood of someone living with HIV, such as through a needle stick

The virus can also be transmitted through a blood transfusion or organ and tissue transplant. However, rigorous testing for HIV among blood, organ, and tissue donors ensures that this is very rare in the United States. It's theoretically possible, but considered extremely rare, for HIV to spread through:

• oral sex (only if there are bleeding gums or open sores in the person's mouth)

• being bitten by a person with HIV (only if the saliva is bloody or there are open sores in the person's mouth)

• contact between broken skin, wounds, or mucous membranes and the blood of someone living with HIV

HIV does NOT spread through:

• skin-to-skin contact

• hugging, shaking hands, or kissing

• air or water

• sharing food or drinks, including drinking fountains

• saliva, tears, or sweat (unless mixed with the blood of a person with HIV)

• sharing a toilet, towels, or bedding

• mosquitoes or other insects

It's important to note that if a person with HIV is being treated and has a persistently undetectable viral load, it's virtually impossible to transmit the virus to another person.

Causes Of HIV

HIV is a variation of a virus that infects African chimpanzees. Scientists suspect the simian immunodeficiency virus (SIV) jumped from chimps to humans when people consumed infected chimpanzee meat. Once inside the human population, the virus mutated into what we now know as HIV. This likely occurred as long ago as the 1920s. HIV spread from person to person throughout Africa over the course of several decades. Eventually, the virus migrated to other parts of the world. Scientists first discovered HIV in a human blood sample in 1959. It's thought that HIV has existed in the United States since the 1970s, but it didn't start to hit public consciousness until the 1980s.

Causes Of AIDS

AIDS is caused by HIV. A person can't get AIDS if they haven't contracted HIV. Healthy individuals have a CD4 count of 500 to 1,500 per cubic millimeter. Without treatment, HIV continues to multiply and destroy CD4 cells. If a person's CD4 count falls below 200, they have AIDS. Also, if someone with HIV develops an opportunistic infection associated with HIV, they can still be diagnosed with AIDS, even if their CD4 count is above 200.

Diagnosis Of HIV

Several different tests can be used to diagnose HIV. Healthcare providers determine which test is best for each person.

Antibody/antigen tests

Antibody/antigen tests are the most commonly used tests. They can show positive results typically within 18–45 days after someone initially contracts HIV. These tests check the blood for antibodies and antigens. An antibody is a type of protein the body makes to fight an infection. An antigen, on the other hand, is the part of the virus that activates the immune system.

Antibody tests

These tests check the blood solely for antibodies. Between 23 and 90 days after transmission, most people will develop detectable HIV antibodies, which can be found in the blood or saliva. These tests are done using blood tests or mouth swabs, and there's no preparation necessary. Some tests provide results in 30 minutes or less and can be performed in a healthcare provider's office or clinic. Other antibody tests can be done at home:

• OraQuick HIV Test. An oral swab provides results in as little as 20 minutes.

• Home Access HIV-1 Test System. After the person pricks their finger, they send a blood sample to a licensed laboratory. They can remain anonymous and call for results the next business day.

If someone suspects they've been exposed to HIV but tested negative in a home test, they should repeat the test in three months. If they have a positive result, they should follow up with their healthcare provider to confirm.

Nucleic acid test (NAT)

This expensive test isn't used for general screening. It's for people who have early symptoms of HIV or have a known risk factor. This test doesn't look for antibodies; it looks for the virus itself. It takes from 5 to 21 days for HIV to be detectable in the blood. This test is usually accompanied or confirmed by an antibody test. Today, it's easier than ever to get tested for HIV.

HIV Window Period

As soon as someone contracts HIV, it starts to reproduce in their body. The person's immune system reacts to the antigens (parts of the virus) by producing antibodies (cells that fight the virus). The time between exposure to HIV and when it becomes detectable in the blood is called the HIV window period. Most people develop detectable HIV antibodies within 23 to 90 days after infection. If a person takes an HIV test during the window period, it's likely they'll receive a negative result. However, they can still transmit the virus to others during this time. If someone thinks they may have been exposed to HIV but tested negative during this time, they should repeat the test in a few months to confirm (the timing depends on the test used). And during that time, they need to use condoms to prevent possibly spreading HIV. Someone who tests negative during the window might benefit from post-exposure prophylaxis (PEP). This is medication taken after an exposure to prevent getting HIV. PEP needs to be taken as soon as possible after the exposure; it should be taken no later than 72 hours after exposure, but ideally before then. Another way to prevent getting HIV is pre-exposure prophylaxis (PrEP). A combination of HIV drugs taken before potential exposure to HIV, PrEP can lower the risk of contracting or spreading HIV when taken consistently. Timing is important when testing for HIV.

Early Symptoms Of HIV

The first few weeks after someone contracts HIV is called the acute infection stage. During this time, the virus reproduces rapidly. The person's immune system responds by producing HIV antibodies. These are proteins that fight infection. During this stage, some people have no symptoms at first. However, many people experience symptoms in the first month or two after contracting the virus, but often don't realize they're caused by HIV. This is because symptoms of the acute stage can be very similar to those of the flu or other seasonal viruses. They may be mild to severe, they may come and go, and they may last anywhere from a few days to several weeks. Early symptoms of HIV can include:

• fever

• chills

• swollen lymph nodes

- general aches and pains

- skin rash

- sore throat

- headache

- nausea

- upset stomach

Because these symptoms are similar to common illnesses like the flu, the person with them might not think they need to see a healthcare provider. And even if they do, their healthcare provider might suspect the flu or mononucleosis and might not even consider HIV. Whether a person has symptoms or not, during this period their viral load is very high. The viral load is the amount of HIV found in the bloodstream. A high viral load means that HIV can be easily transmitted to someone else during this time. Initial HIV symptoms usually resolve within a few months as the person enters the chronic, or clinical latency, stage of HIV. This stage can last many years or even decades with treatment. HIV symptoms can vary from person to person.

Symptoms Of HIV

After the first month or so, HIV enters the clinical latency stage. This stage can last from a few years to a few decades. Some people don't have any symptoms during this time, while others may have minimal or nonspecific symptoms. A nonspecific symptom is a symptom that doesn't pertain to one specific disease or condition. These nonspecific symptoms may include:

• headaches and other aches and pains

• swollen lymph nodes

• recurrent fevers

• night sweats

• fatigue

• nausea

• vomiting

• diarrhea

• weight loss

• skin rashes

• recurrent oral or vaginal yeast infections

• pneumonia

• shingles

As with the early stage, HIV is still infectious during this time even without symptoms and can be transmitted to another person. However, a person won't know they have HIV unless they get tested. If someone has these symptoms and thinks they may have been exposed to HIV, it's important that they get tested. HIV symptoms at this stage may come and go, or they may progress rapidly. This progression can be slowed substantially with treatment. With the consistent use of this antiretroviral therapy, chronic HIV can last for decades and will likely not develop into AIDS, if treatment was started early enough.

Is rash a symptom of HIV?

About 90 percent of people with HIV experience changes to their skin. Rash is often one of the first symptoms of HIV infection. Generally, an HIV rash appears as multiple small red lesions that are flat and raised.

Rash related to HIV: HIV makes someone more susceptible to skin problems because the virus destroys immune system cells that fight infection. Co-infections that can cause rash include:

• molluscum contagiosum

• herpes simplex

• shingles

The appearance of the rash, how long it lasts, and how it can be treated depends on the cause.

Rash related to medication: While rash can be caused by HIV co-infections, it can also be caused by medication. Some drugs used to treat HIV or other infections can cause a rash. This type of rash usually appears within a week or two of starting a new medication. Sometimes the rash will clear up on its own. If it doesn't, a change in medications may be needed. Rash due to an allergic reaction to medication can be serious. Other symptoms of an allergic reaction include trouble breathing or swallowing, dizziness, and fever. Stevens-Johnson syndrome (SJS) is a rare allergic reaction to HIV medication. Symptoms include fever and swelling of the face and tongue. A blistering rash, which can involve the skin and mucous membranes, appears and spreads quickly. When 30 percent of the skin is affected it's called toxic epidermal necrolysis, which is a life-threatening condition. If this develops, emergency medical care is needed. While rash can be linked with HIV or HIV medications, it's important to keep in mind that rashes are common and can have many other causes.

HIV symptoms in men

Symptoms of HIV vary from person to person, but they're similar in men and women. These symptoms can come and go or get progressively worse. If a person has been exposed to HIV, they may also have been exposed to other sexually transmitted infections (STIs). These include gonorrhea, chlamydia, syphilis, and trichomoniasis. Men may be more likely than women to notice symptoms of STIs such as sores on their genitals. However, men typically don't seek medical care as often as women.

HIV symptoms in women

For the most part, symptoms of HIV are similar in men and women. However, symptoms they experience overall may differ based on the different risks men and women face if they have HIV. Both men and women with HIV are at increased risk of sexually transmitted infections (STIs). However, women may be less likely than men to notice small spots or other changes to their genitals. In addition, women with HIV are at increased risk of:

• recurrent vaginal yeast infections

• other vaginal infections, including bacterial vaginosis

• pelvic inflammatory disease (PID)

• menstrual cycle changes

• human papillomavirus (HPV), which can cause genital warts and lead to cervical cancer

While not related to HIV symptoms, another risk for women with HIV is that the virus can be transmitted to a baby during pregnancy. However, antiretroviral therapy is considered safe during pregnancy. Women who are treated with antiretroviral therapy are at very low risk of passing HIV to their baby during pregnancy and delivery. Breastfeeding is also affected in women with HIV. The virus can be passed to a baby through breast milk. In the United States and other settings where formula is accessible and safe, it's recommended that women with HIV not breastfeed their babies. For these women, use of formula is encouraged. Options besides formula include pasteurized banked human milk. For women who may have been exposed to HIV, it's important to know what symptoms to look for.

Symptoms Of AIDS

AIDS refers to acquired immunodeficiency syndrome. With this condition, the immune system is weakened due to HIV that's typically gone untreated for many years. If HIV is found and treated early with antiretroviral therapy, a person will usually not develop AIDS. People with HIV may develop AIDS if their HIV is not diagnosed until late, or if they know they have HIV but don't consistently take their antiretroviral therapy. They may also develop AIDS if they have a type of HIV that's resistant to (doesn't respond to) the antiretroviral treatment. Without proper and consistent treatment, people living with HIV can develop AIDS sooner. By that time, the immune system is quite damaged and has a harder time fighting off infection and disease. With the use of antiretroviral therapy, a person can maintain chronic HIV infection without developing AIDS for decades. Symptoms of AIDS can include:

• recurrent fever

- chronic swollen lymph glands, especially of the armpits, neck, and groin

- chronic fatigue

- night sweats

- dark splotches under the skin or inside the mouth, nose, or eyelids

- sores, spots, or lesions of the mouth and tongue, genitals, or anus

- bumps, lesions, or rashes of the skin

- recurrent or chronic diarrhea

- rapid weight loss

- neurologic problems such as trouble concentrating, memory loss, and confusion

- anxiety and depression

Antiretroviral therapy controls the virus and usually prevents progression to AIDS. Other infections and complications of AIDS can also be treated. That treatment must be tailored to the individual needs of the person.

Treatment Options For HIV

Treatment should begin as soon as possible after a diagnosis of HIV, regardless of viral load. The main treatment for HIV is antiretroviral therapy, a combination of daily medications that stop the virus from reproducing. This helps protect CD4 cells, keeping the immune system strong enough to fight off disease. Antiretroviral therapy helps keep HIV from progressing to AIDS. It also helps reduce the risk of transmitting HIV to others. When treatment is effective, the viral load will be "undetectable." The person still has HIV, but the virus is not visible in test results. However, the virus is still in the body. And if that person stops taking antiretroviral therapy, the viral load will increase again and the HIV can again start attacking CD4 cells.

HIV Medications

More than 25 antiretroviral therapy medications are approved to treat HIV. They work to prevent HIV from reproducing and destroying CD4 cells, which help the immune system fight infection. This helps reduce the risk of developing complications related to HIV, as well as transmitting the virus to others. These antiretroviral medications are grouped into six classes:

• nucleoside reverse transcriptase inhibitors (NRTIs)

• non-nucleoside reverse transcriptase inhibitors (NNRTIs)

• protease inhibitors

• fusion inhibitors

• CCR5 antagonists, also known as entry inhibitors

• integrase strand transfer inhibitors

Treatment regimens

The U.S. Department of Health and Human Services (HHS) generally recommends a starting regimen of three HIV medications from at least two of these drug classes. This combination helps prevent HIV from forming resistance to medications. (Resistance means the drug no longer works to treat the virus.) Many of the antiretroviral medications are combined with others so that a person with HIV typically takes only one or two pills a day. A healthcare provider will help a person with HIV choose a regimen based on their overall health and personal circumstances.

These medications must be taken every day, exactly as prescribed. If they're not taken appropriately, viral resistance can develop, and a new regimen may be needed. Blood testing will help determine if the regimen is working to keep the viral load down and the CD4 count up. If an antiretroviral therapy regimen isn't working, the person's healthcare provider will switch them to a different regimen that's more effective.

Side effects and costs

Side effects of antiretroviral therapy vary and may include nausea, headache, and dizziness. These symptoms are often temporary and disappear with time. Serious side effects can include swelling of the mouth and tongue and liver or kidney damage. If side effects are severe, the medications can be adjusted. Costs for antiretroviral therapy vary according to geographic location and type of insurance coverage. Some pharmaceutical companies have assistance programs to help lower the cost.

HIV Prevention

Although many researchers are working to develop one, there's currently no vaccine available to prevent the transmission of HIV. However, taking certain steps can help prevent the spread of HIV.

Safer sex

The most common way for HIV to spread is through anal or vaginal sex without a condom. This risk can't be completely eliminated unless sex is avoided entirely, but the risk can be lowered considerably by taking a few precautions. A person concerned about their risk of HIV should:

• Get tested for HIV. It's important they learn their status and that of their partner.

• Get tested for other sexually transmitted infections (STIs). If they test positive for one, they should get it treated, because having an STI increases the risk of contracting HIV.

• Use condoms. They should learn the correct way to use condoms and use them every time they have sex, whether it's through vaginal or anal intercourse. It's important to keep in mind that pre-seminal fluids (which come out before male ejaculation) can contain HIV.

• Limit their sexual partners. They should have one sexual partner with whom they have an exclusive sexual relationship.

• Take their medications as directed if they have HIV. This lowers the risk of transmitting the virus to their sexual partner.

Other prevention methods
Other steps to help prevent the spread of HIV include:

• Avoid sharing needles or other drug paraphernalia. HIV is transmitted through blood and can be contracted by using contaminated materials.

• Consider PEP. A person who has been exposed to HIV should contact their healthcare provider about obtaining post-exposure prophylaxis (PEP). PEP can reduce the risk of contracting HIV. It consists of three antiretroviral medications given for 28 days. PEP should be started as soon as possible after exposure, but before 36 to 72 hours have passed.

• Consider PrEP. A person at a high risk of HIV should talk to their healthcare provider about pre-exposure prophylaxis (PrEP). If taken consistently, it can lower the risk of contracting HIV. PrEP is a combination of two drugs available in pill form.

Healthcare providers can offer more information on these and other ways to prevent the spread of HIV.

Living With HIV

More than 1 million people in the United States are living with HIV. It's different for everybody, but with treatment, many can expect to live a long, productive life. The most important thing is to start antiretroviral treatment as soon as possible. By taking medications exactly as prescribed, people living with HIV can keep their viral load low and their immune system strong. It's also important to follow up with a healthcare provider regularly. Other ways people living with HIV can improve their health include:

Make their health their top priority. Steps to help people living with HIV feel their best include:

• fueling their body with a well-balanced diet

• exercising regularly

• getting plenty of rest

• avoiding tobacco and other drugs

• reporting any new symptoms to their healthcare provider right away

Focus on their emotional health. They could consider seeing a licensed therapist who is experienced in treating people with HIV.

Use safer sex practices. Talk to their sexual partner(s). Get tested for other sexually transmitted infections (STIs). And use condoms every time they have vaginal or anal sex.

Talk to their healthcare provider about PrEP and PEP. When used consistently by a person without HIV, pre-exposure prophylaxis (PrEP) and post-exposure prophylaxis (PEP) can lower the chances of transmission. PrEP is most often recommended for people without HIV in relationships with people with HIV, but it can be used in other situations as well. Online sources for finding a PrEP provider include PrEP Locator and PleasePrEPMe.

Surround themselves with loved ones. When first telling people about their diagnosis, they can start slow by telling someone who can maintain their confidence. They may want to choose someone who won't judge them, and who will support them in caring for their health.

Get support. They can join an HIV support group, either in person or online, so they can meet with others who face the same concerns they have. And their healthcare provider can steer them toward a variety of resources in their area.

There are many ways to get the most out of life when living with HIV.

HIV Life Expectancy

In the 1990s, a 20-year-old person with HIV had a 19-year life expectancy. By 2011, a 20-year-old person with HIV could expect to live another 53 years. It's a dramatic improvement, due in large part to antiretroviral therapy. With proper treatment, many people with HIV can expect a normal or near normal lifespan. Of course, many things affect life expectancy for a person with HIV. Among them are:

• CD4 cell count

• viral load

• serious HIV-related illnesses, including hepatitis infection

• drug use

• smoking

• access, adherence, and response to treatment

• other health conditions

• age

Where a person lives also matters. People in the United States and other developed countries may be more likely to have access to antiretroviral therapy. Consistent use of these drugs helps prevent HIV from progressing to AIDS. When HIV advances to AIDS, life expectancy without treatment is about three years. In 2017, about 20.9 million people living with HIV were using antiretroviral therapy. Life expectancy statistics are just general guidelines. People living with HIV should talk to their healthcare provider to learn more about what they can expect.

Vaccine For HIV

Currently, there are no vaccines to prevent or treat HIV. Research and testing on experimental vaccines are ongoing, but none are close to being approved for general use. HIV is a complicated virus. It mutates (changes) rapidly and is often able to fend off immune system responses. Only a small number of people who have HIV develop broadly neutralizing antibodies, the kind of antibodies that can fight a range of HIV strains. The first HIV vaccine efficacy study in seven years is currently underway in South Africa. The experimental vaccine is an updated version of one used in a 2009 trial that took place in Thailand. A 3.5-year follow-up after vaccination showed the vaccine was 31.2 percent effective in preventing HIV infection. It's the most successful HIV vaccine trial to date. The study involves 5,400 men and women from South Africa. In 2016 in South Africa, about 270,000 people contracted HIV. The results of the study are expected in 2021. While there's still no vaccine to prevent HIV, people with HIV can benefit from other vaccines to prevent HIV-related illnesses, such as:

• pneumonia

• influenza

• hepatitis A and B

• meningitis

• shingles

Other research into an HIV vaccine is also ongoing.

HIV Statistics

Here are today's HIV numbers:

• In 2016, about 36.7 million people worldwide were living with HIV. Of those, 2.1 million were children below the age of 15.

• In 2017, only 20.9 million people living with HIV were using antiretroviral therapy.

• Since the pandemic began, 76.1 million people have contracted HIV, and AIDS-related complications have claimed 35 million lives.

• In 2016, 1 million people died from AIDS-related diseases. This is a decline from 1.9 million in 2005.

• Eastern and southern Africa are hardest hit. In 2016, 19.4 million people in these areas were living with HIV, and 790,000 more contracted the virus. The region has more than half of all people living with HIV worldwide.

• Every 9.5 minutes, someone in the United States contracts the virus. That's more than 56,000 new cases a year. It's estimated that 1.1 million Americans are currently living with HIV, and 1 in 5 don't know that they have it.

• About 180,000 American women are living with HIV. In the United States, almost half of all new cases occur in African-Americans.

• Untreated, a woman with HIV has a 25 percent chance of passing HIV to her baby during pregnancy or breastfeeding. With antiretroviral therapy throughout pregnancy and avoidance of breastfeeding, the risk is less than 2 percent.

• In the 1990s, a 20-year-old person with HIV had a life expectancy of 19 years. By 2011, it had improved to 53 years. Today, life expectancy is near normal if antiretroviral therapy is started soon after contracting HIV.

As access to antiretroviral therapy continues to improve around the world, these statistics will hopefully keep changing.

Herpes

Herpes simplex is a virus. That means that there isn't a known "cure" that will prevent symptoms from returning. But there are things you can do to find relief during an HSV-1 or HSV-2 outbreak. You may be able to reduce inflammation, irritation, and other symptoms through a mix of lifestyle changes and dietary supplements. However, these remedies aren't a replacement for a clinical treatment plan.

Herpes Simplex

The herpes simplex virus, also known as HSV, is an infection that causes herpes. Herpes can appear in various parts of the body, most commonly on the genitals or mouth. There are two types of the herpes simplex virus.

• HSV-1: primarily causes oral herpes, and is generally responsible for cold sores and fever blisters around the mouth and on the face.

• HSV-2: primarily causes genital herpes, and is generally responsible for genital herpes outbreaks.

Causes Of Herpes Simplex

The herpes simplex virus is a contagious virus that can be transmitted from person to person through direct contact. Children will often contract HSV-1 from early contact with an infected adult. They then carry the virus with them for the rest of their lives.

HSV-1

HSV-1 can be contracted from general interactions such as:

• eating from the same utensils

• sharing lip balm

• kissing

The virus spreads more quickly when an infected person is experiencing an outbreak. An estimated 67 percent of people ages 49 or younger are seropositive for HSV-1, though they may never experience an outbreak. It's also possible to get genital herpes from HSV-1 if someone who performed oral sex had cold sores during that time.

HSV-2

HSV-2 is contracted through forms of sexual contact with a person who has HSV-2. An estimated 20 percent of sexually active adults in the United States are infected with HSV-2, according to the American Academy of Dermatology (AAD). HSV-2 infections are spread through contact with a herpes sore. In contrast, most people get HSV-1 from an infected person who is asymptomatic, or does not have sores.

Risk Of Developing Herpes Simplex Infections

Anyone can be infected with HSV, regardless of age. Your risk is based almost entirely on exposure to the infection. In cases of sexually transmitted HSV, people are more at risk when they have sex not protected by condoms or other barrier methods. Other risk factors for HSV-2 include:

• having multiple sex partners

• having sex at a younger age

• being female

• having another sexually transmitted infection (STI)

• having a weakened immune system

If a pregnant woman is having an outbreak of genital herpes at the time of childbirth, it can expose the baby to both types of HSV, and may put them at risk for serious complications.

Recognizing The Signs Of Herpes Simplex

It's important to understand that someone may not have visible sores or symptoms and still be infected by the virus. They may also transmit the virus to others. Some of the symptoms associated with this virus include:

• blistering sores (in the mouth or on the genitals)

• pain during urination (genital herpes)

• itching

You may also experience symptoms that are similar to the flu. These symptoms can include:

• fever

• swollen lymph nodes

• headaches

• tiredness

• lack of appetite

HSV can also spread to the eyes, causing a condition called herpes keratitis. This can cause symptoms such as eye pain, discharge, and a gritty feeling in the eye.

Herpes Simplex Diagnosis

This type of virus is generally diagnosed with a physical exam. Your doctor may check your body for sores and ask you about some of your symptoms. Your doctor may also request HSV testing. This is known as a herpes culture. It will confirm the diagnosis if you have sores on your genitals. During this test, your doctor will take a swab sample of fluid from the sore and then send it to a laboratory for testing. Blood tests for antibodies to HSV-1 and HSV-2 can also help diagnose these infections. This is especially helpful when there are no sores present.

Herpes Simplex Treatment

There is currently no cure for this virus. Treatment focuses on getting rid of sores and limiting outbreaks. It's possible that your sores will go away without treatment. However, your doctor may determine you need one or more of the following medications:

• acyclovir

• famciclovir

• valacyclovir

These medications can help people infected with the virus reduce the risk of transmitting it to others. The medications also help to lower the intensity and frequency of outbreaks. These medications may come in oral (pill) form, or may be applied as a cream. For severe outbreaks, these medications may also be administered by injection.

Long-Term Outlook For Herpes Simplex

People who become infected with HSV will have the virus for the rest of their lives. Even if it does not manifest symptoms, the virus will continue to live in an infected person's nerve cells. Some people may experience regular outbreaks. Others will only experience one outbreak after they have been infected and then the virus may become dormant. Even if a virus is dormant, certain stimuli can trigger an outbreak. These include:

• stress

• menstrual periods

• fever or illness

• sun exposure or sunburn

It's believed that outbreaks may become less intense over time because the body starts creating antibodies. If a generally healthy person is infected with the virus, there are usually no complications.

Preventing The Spread Of Herpes Simplex Infections
Although there is no cure for herpes, you can take measures to avoid contracting the virus, or to prevent transmitting

HSV to another person. If you're experiencing an outbreak of HSV-1, consider taking a few preventive steps:

• Try to avoid direct physical contact with other people.

• Don't share any items that can pass the virus around, such as cups, towels, silverware, clothing, makeup, or lip balm.

• Don't participate in oral sex, kissing, or any other type of sexual activity during an outbreak.

• Wash your hands thoroughly and apply medication with cotton swabs to reduce contact with sores.

People with HSV-2 should avoid any type of sexual activity with other people during an outbreak. If the person is not experiencing symptoms but has been diagnosed with the virus, a condom should be used during intercourse. But even when using a condom, the virus can still be passed to a partner from uncovered skin. Women who are pregnant and infected may have to take medication to prevent the virus from infecting their unborn babies.

Dr. Sebi Cure For HIV And Herpes

Dr. Sebi And AIDS

The recent killing of American rapper Nipsey Hussle sparked fresh interest in a controversial self-proclaimed natural healer Alfredo Bowman, popularly known as Dr Sebi. According to social media conspiracy theorists and sleuths, Hussle was gunned down on March 31, 2019, to thwart his plans to produce a documentary profiling the life of Dr Sebi and how he had cured AIDS and other ailments using herbal remedies. Before his demise, Hussle was reportedly working on a documentary on the Honduran herbalist, who in 1985 beat a New York court case for claiming he could cure AIDS. Dr Sebi had run ads in various newspapers and magazines saying that "AIDs has been cured". For an initial payment of $500 (Sh 50,000) and $800 (Sh 80,000) for subsequent visits, Dr Sebi claimed that he could cure his patients of AIDS and other ailments including diabetes, sickle cell anaemia, lupus, herpes, and cancer. The self-taught intracellular therapist and herbalist prescribed a strict raw vegan diet that also cut out alcohol, sugar, and salt to help body cells heal and regenerate. "I am working on doing a documentary on the trial in 1985," Nipsey Hussle said in an interview. "When

Dr Sebi went to trial in New York because he put in the newspaper that he cured AIDs. He beat that case. But nobody talks about it. I think the story is important." After winning the case, Dr Sebi went on to work with various celebrities, including Michael Jackson, Steven Seagal, Eddie Murphy, John Travolta, and Lisa "Left Eye" Lopez. Lisa Lopez even showed public support for Dr Sebi by proclaiming "I know a man who has been curing AIDS since 1987." Shortly afterwards, Lopez was run off the road and killed after leaving Dr Sebi's Usha Healing Village in Honduras. Conspiracy theorists believe she was also targeted because of spreading Dr Sebi's healing message. Dr Sebi is said to have worked with Michael Jackson to treat his addiction to painkillers. He later sued the King of Pop $380,000 in unpaid bills and $600,000 in lost revenue. The case was dismissed in 2015 due to lack of prosecution. Born in 1933 in Honduras, Dr Sebi moved to the United States at the age of 20 and started marketing his herbal products in the 1980s. He claimed that he had been diagnosed with asthma, diabetes, impotency and obesity. He managed to cure himself of all these ailments with herbal medicine, after years of unsuccessful treatment with conventional western medicine. Inspired by his personal healing, he delved into the world of natural medicine. He dedicated over 30 years of his life to creating natural vegetation cell food compounds aimed at intra-cellular cleansing and revitalisation. He later founded the USHA Research Institute, and USHA Healing Village in his home country to promote natural healing. Dr Sebi died at the age of 82 in a Honduran jail cell in 2016 after he was arrested for carrying huge sums of money. Although the official cause of death was penned down as pneumonia, some think that the herbal guru was murdered by the medical industry to silence his message.

Dr Sebi's food principles

Dr Sebi grouped foods into six categories: live, raw, dead, hybrid, genetically modified or drugs. He insisted that for one to be healthy, they needed to feed on only foods in the first two categories, which he termed as "electric foods." These foods, Dr Sebi claimed, were alkaline in nature and could heal body from effects caused by foods in the latter categories. He made a list of alkaline foods which includes plain ripe fruit, non-starchy vegetables such as leafy greens, raw nuts and nut butters, and grains such as quinoa, amaranth (terere), rye, kamut, and wild rice. Dead and acidic foods, on the other hand include all types of meat, poultry, seafood, products containing leavening agents such as yeast, alcohol, sugar, iodized salt, processed foods, and any fried food. Adherents to Dr Sebi's diet plan are also advised to avoid seedless fruits, insect or weather resistant crops such as corn, and anything fortified with added vitamins and minerals.

Dr Sebi believed that there was only one disease a body could have, only that it manifested differently. "There's only one disease: compromised mucous membranes," he's widely reported to have said. His website dissects Western medicine thus: "According to Western medical research, diseases are a result of the host being infected with a 'germ', 'virus', or bacteria. "Dr Sebi's had a different approach. "We examine the African approach to disease; it diametrically opposes the present Western approach. Specifically, the African Bio-mineral Balance refutes the germ/virus/bacteria premise. Our research reveals that all manifestation of disease finds its genesis when and where the mucous membrane has been compromised." The benefits of eating a vegan/vegetarian diet are undeniable- it can significantly reduce risk of cancer, heart disease, type 2 diabetes, high blood pressure, and elevated blood cholesterol. However, note that the alkaline diet has been scientifically discredited. Studies have found that while what you eat can affect the acidity of your urine, there's very little change in blood pH. Robert Young, a doctor who's widely credited for creating the alkaline diet was convicted for having bought his doctorate from a correspondence school. Because Dr Sebi's diet greatly reduces or eliminates whole groups of food, strict adherents might also experience deficiencies in essential nutrients such as iron, calcium, vitamin D, Vitamin B12, and omega 3 fatty acids. It's therefore advisable to load up on supplements. There is no research to support Dr Sebi's theory that mucous cleansing can cure disease. Dr Sebi wasn't medically trained and only offered anecdotal evidence for his claims, not well-documented clinical tests. Dr Sebi's diet can also be quite limiting, making it difficult to eat out or enjoy eating with family and friends.

Dr Sebi Herpes Cure

Cleanse your body, starve the parasites, replenish the cells that were previously damaged.

• Herbs to Take: Replenish the Iron in Your Body with Iron Plus & Bio Ferro

• Fasting: Try to fast as much as possible

• Foods to Eat: Follow the Dr Sebi Nutritional Guide, but place a large focus on green leafy vegetables. Bitter foods are better to eat in this situation and you should only consume minimal amounts of fruits and vegetables that are sweet.

• Foods not to Eat: Stay away from acidic foods, especially starches and sweets which feed parasites. Also do not eat chickpeas, avocados, and quinoa while treating even though they are on the nutritional guide.

How Long Does It Take To Get Rid Of Herpes

Dr Sebi was once asked how long should a person cleans and detox and I think that the answer that Dr Sebi gave applies to this question. If you have plant-based iron teas such as burdock, dandelion, yellow dock, this will help. Consume them several times a day for as long a period as you can; ten days minimum. You do not have to mix them. If you would like to, that is your choice. They may be difficult to find depending on where you are. You may have to order the roots from online herbal websites. Practice fasting; plan and go for it. The more you fast the quicker you heal. If you feel weak, eat dates. They are sweet but shouldn't agitate your cells. Only eat them when you feel weak. Eat salads as if you were eating a bag of potato chips. Get the light crisp kind, but no iceberg salad. The answer according to what Dr. Sebi teaches is to get rid of the mucus in the body, and it goes like this: There is only one disease and that is the result of the mucous membrane being compromised. The mucous membrane is necessary to maintain health because it is the membrane that protects the cells. When you break the mucous membrane down it turns to pus and expose the cells. For example, Sickle Cell Anemia is when the blood plasma has broken down by mucous into a sickle. Mucous sinks into the plasma, into the cell itself, breaks and disunites the cell. Removing the mucous the cell unites again. To maintain that level, you have to feed the patient large doses of iron phosphate. Not ferrous oxide. The Iron based herbal compounds produced by Dr. Sebi such as the Iron Plus and Bio Ferro, provides your body with over 14 key organic (carbon-hydrogen-oxygen) plant and herb based minerals. The suite of vegetation cell food products not only contain Iron Phosphate, they are derived from electrically charged tropical plants and herbs; some of which come from tropical Africa, Honduras, the Caribbean, other Latin American countries and the United States. The plants and herbs contained in Dr. Sebi's vegetation cell food compounds are highly electrical. Their molecular structure is complete and carbon-based. They will immediately assimilate and energize the body with the food provided for us by nature. The compounds, provides you with necessary phosphates, carbonates, iodides and bromides…The Food of Life!